AEROBICS FOR SENIORS

Aerobic Exercises That Are Easy To Follow And Promote Heart Health,

Endurance, And Energy Levels.

Basil U

COPYRIGHT

TABLE OF CONTENTS

ABOUT THE BOOK

As we navigate the journey of aging, maintaining physical health becomes increasingly important. "Aerobics for Seniors" serves as a comprehensive guide designed specifically for older adults seeking to enhance their health and well-being through safe and enjoyable aerobic exercises. This book recognizes the unique needs and challenges faced by seniors, offering tailored solutions that promote heart health, build endurance, and boost energy levels all while ensuring that exercises are easy to follow and adaptable to various fitness levels.

The Importance of Aerobic Exercise for Seniors

Aerobic exercise is vital for seniors for several reasons. Regular physical activity helps combat the natural decline in cardiovascular health that occurs with age. It can improve circulation, lower blood pressure, and reduce the risk of heart disease, all of which are critical considerations for older adults. Furthermore, engaging in aerobic activities fosters endurance, allowing seniors to perform daily activities with greater ease and less fatigue. This not only enhances quality of life but also promotes independence.

In addition to the physical benefits, aerobic exercises have a profound impact on mental and emotional well-being. Many seniors experience feelings of isolation or depression, but staying active can significantly alleviate these feelings by releasing endorphins, improving mood, and fostering social connections. This book emphasizes the holistic benefits of aerobics, encouraging readers to view fitness not just as a physical endeavor but as a pathway to improved mental and emotional health.

Tailored Content for Senior Readers

Understanding that seniors may have varying levels of physical ability and fitness experience, "Aerobics for Seniors" is structured to cater to all fitness levels. The book is divided into chapters that cover essential topics related to senior-friendly aerobics, including:

- Understanding Aerobic Exercise: A foundational overview of what aerobic exercise entails, its benefits, and how it differs from other forms of exercise.
- Getting Started: Guidance on assessing fitness levels, consulting with healthcare providers, and setting realistic goals to ensure a safe start.
- Safe and Easy-to-Follow Aerobic Exercises: A detailed exploration of low-impact activities such as walking aerobics, chair workouts, water aerobics, and even dancing, all designed to promote heart health while being gentle on the joints.
- Building Endurance: Strategies for gradually increasing the intensity of workouts, the long-term benefits of improved stamina, and tips to avoid burnout.
- Energy-Boosting Workouts: Short-burst exercises that combat fatigue, promote better sleep, and improve mood, along with nutritional advice to sustain energy during workouts.
- Group Aerobic Classes: The social benefits of exercising with others, how to find or create local groups, and the growing availability of online aerobic classes.
- Adapting Exercises for Chronic Conditions: Practical advice for seniors with arthritis, diabetes, osteoporosis, and other chronic conditions, ensuring that everyone can participate safely and effectively.
- Home Workouts: Tips for designing a home-based aerobic routine, including minimal equipment exercises and the incorporation of technology through fitness apps and online videos.
- Motivation and Overcoming Barriers: Strategies to combat common excuses, maintain motivation, set realistic goals, and celebrate the rewards of regular aerobic exercise.

A Storytelling Approach to Engage Readers

"Aerobics for Seniors" is written in a modern, accessible style, incorporating storytelling elements to keep readers engaged. Each chapter is interwoven with personal anecdotes and success stories from seniors who have transformed their lives through aerobic activity. These narratives serve not only as inspiration but also as relatable examples of the challenges and triumphs encountered on the journey to fitness. Readers will find themselves immersed in stories of resilience, camaraderie, and the sheer joy of movement.

Practical Advice and Resources

Throughout the book, practical advice is provided in a clear and straightforward manner, ensuring that seniors can easily implement the recommendations into their daily lives. The appendices offer valuable resources, including sample workout plans, exercises for those with mobility challenges, a heart rate chart, and a directory for finding local and online senior aerobic classes.

A Call to Action for Lifelong Fitness

Ultimately, "Aerobics for Seniors" is more than just a fitness manual; it is a call to action for seniors to embrace the joy of movement and prioritize their health. The book encourages readers to view aerobic exercise as a lifelong commitment, an essential part of a vibrant and fulfilling life. Whether you're just starting your fitness journey or looking to enhance your existing routine, this book offers the tools, motivation, and community support needed to thrive.

As you turn the pages of "Aerobics for Seniors," you'll discover that it's never too late to start moving, and the benefits of aerobic exercise extend far beyond physical fitness; they encompass a richer, more engaged, and healthier life.

INTRODUCTION

As we age, the rhythms of life often shift. The bustling energy of youth gives way to a slower pace, and our bodies can begin to feel the weight of years gone by. Yet, amidst this transition lies a powerful truth: staying active is one of the most vital keys to aging gracefully. Aerobics, in particular, offers a dynamic avenue for seniors to reclaim their vitality and enhance their quality of life.

Aerobic exercises are not just about breaking a sweat; they represent a cornerstone of healthy living for older adults. Engaging in regular aerobic activity can help improve cardiovascular health, boost endurance, and elevate energy levels. Imagine a gentle morning walk that not only lifts your spirits but also strengthens your heart, or a fun dance class that leaves you invigorated. These activities foster a sense of community, create joyful moments, and remind us that movement can be a celebration, not just a routine.

At the heart of aerobic exercise lies its profound impact on our bodies. As we engage in activities that elevate our heart rate, we promote blood circulation, which in turn nourishes our organs and tissues. This increased circulation can enhance our overall physical health, reduce the risk of chronic illnesses, and even improve cognitive function. It's a win-win for both body and mind.

Moreover, the benefits of aerobic exercises extend beyond just the physical. They play a crucial role in boosting endurance, allowing seniors to participate more fully in daily activities whether it's playing with grandchildren, gardening, or simply enjoying a leisurely stroll. Increased energy levels can significantly improve mood, fostering a sense of empowerment and positivity that permeates all aspects of life.

This book is designed to guide you through the world of senior aerobics, offering practical advice, simple routines, and inspiring success stories. With a focus on adapting exercises to fit individual needs and capabilities, we aim to make aerobic activities accessible to everyone. By weaving together personal anecdotes and relatable insights, we hope to create an engaging narrative that encourages you to embrace the joy of movement.

So, let's embark on this journey together. It's time to rediscover the joy of staying active and to unlock the many benefits that aerobic exercise can bring. The path to a healthier, more energetic life is just a few steps away.

CHAPTER 1

UNDERSTANDING SENIOR-FRIENDLY AEROBICS

Aerobic exercise: what does that really mean? At its core, aerobic exercise refers to any physical activity that raises your heart rate and gets your blood pumping. This includes a variety of activities such as walking, swimming, cycling, dancing, and even gardening. The term "aerobic" comes from the Greek word for "oxygen," which emphasizes the role that this vital element plays in fueling our muscles during exercise.

For seniors, incorporating aerobic activities into their routine is essential for maintaining overall health and vitality. As we age, our bodies undergo changes that can make us more susceptible to various health issues. Aerobic exercise is a natural, effective way to combat these challenges and promote a better quality of life.

How Aerobic Exercises Improve Cardiovascular Health

One of the most significant benefits of aerobic exercise is its ability to improve cardiovascular health. Regular aerobic activity strengthens the heart, enabling it to pump blood more efficiently throughout the body. This increased efficiency leads to lower blood pressure and improved circulation, reducing the risk of heart disease, a condition that disproportionately affects older adults.

Consider the story of Frank, an 82-year-old retiree who spent most of his days sitting in front of the television. He began to experience fatigue during simple tasks like climbing stairs or playing with his grandchildren. After a visit to his doctor, he learned about the importance of aerobic exercise for his heart health. Encouraged, Frank started walking around his neighborhood for just 20 minutes each day. Over time, he noticed not only an improvement in his endurance but also a remarkable boost in his overall energy levels.

He could once again enjoy playing catch with his grandkids, all because he made a simple change to his routine.

But the benefits don't stop at the heart. Aerobic exercises also promote better lung capacity, ensuring that seniors can take in more oxygen, which is crucial for maintaining stamina. Improved lung function means that seniors can engage in daily activities with greater ease, making it easier to enjoy life's simple pleasures.

Adapting Exercises for Seniors: What's Different?

When we talk about aerobic exercise for seniors, it's crucial to recognize that adaptation is key. As our bodies age, factors such as reduced muscle mass, joint stiffness, and balance issues can impact our ability to perform certain activities. This doesn't mean that seniors should shy away from exercise; rather, it means that modifications can make these activities more accessible and enjoyable.

For example, while high-impact exercises like running or jumping can be invigorating for younger individuals, they might not be suitable for seniors. Instead, options like brisk walking, low-impact aerobics, or cycling offer similar cardiovascular benefits without the risk of injury. These modifications can make all the difference in maintaining motivation and reducing the likelihood of discomfort.

Take the example of Grace, a 70-year-old who loved to dance in her youth. She was eager to get back to her roots but was concerned about her ability to keep up with the fast-paced classes she remembered. Instead of giving up on her passion, Grace found a local senior dance aerobics class tailored to her needs. The instructor modified the routines to ensure they were safe, engaging, and fun, allowing Grace to dance at her own pace. The joy of movement returned to her life, and she formed lasting friendships with others in the class who shared her love for dance.

Importance of Low-Impact and Joint-Friendly Movements

For many seniors, joint health becomes a primary concern, particularly for those who may have arthritis or other mobility issues. High-impact exercises can exacerbate discomfort, making it vital to prioritize low-impact options that are kinder to the joints. Low-impact aerobic exercises allow seniors to reap the benefits of cardiovascular training while minimizing strain on their bodies.

Activities like swimming or water aerobics are excellent examples of low-impact workouts. The buoyancy of the water supports the body, reducing the risk of injury while still providing resistance for a great workout. Similarly, chair aerobics offer an excellent alternative for those with limited mobility, allowing participants to engage in rhythmic movements while seated.

Samantha, a spirited 75-year-old, struggled with knee pain that kept her from enjoying her regular walks in the park. Frustrated but determined, she sought out a local water aerobics class. The first time she submerged herself in the pool, she felt liberated, the water embraced her, and she could move freely without the pressure on her joints. Not only did she find relief from her pain, but she also discovered a supportive community of fellow participants who encouraged each other to stay active.

Low-impact, joint-friendly movements are not just safe; they can also foster a sense of confidence and accomplishment. As seniors gradually build strength and endurance through these exercises, they often find themselves more willing to explore new activities and engage in social opportunities, enhancing their overall well-being.

In summary, understanding aerobic exercise and its adaptations for seniors is essential for cultivating a fulfilling, active lifestyle. By recognizing the unique needs of older adults, we can unlock the transformative benefits of aerobic activities. Improved cardiovascular health, increased endurance, and a focus on low-impact movements all contribute to a more vibrant life.

As we move forward in this book, you'll discover a variety of aerobic exercises tailored specifically for seniors, along with practical tips and inspiring stories that will motivate you to embark on your own fitness journey. Let's take the next step together, celebrating the joy of movement and the possibilities it holds for a healthier future.

CHAPTER 2

GETTING STARTED WITH AEROBICS FOR SENIORS

Embarking on a new fitness journey can be both exciting and intimidating, especially for seniors. Understanding where to start and how to assess your readiness for aerobics is essential for success. This chapter will guide you through assessing your fitness level, the importance of consulting with a doctor, warming up properly, avoiding common pitfalls, and enhancing mobility and flexibility to prepare for aerobic activities.

How to Assess Your Fitness Level

Before diving into any new exercise regimen, it's crucial to assess your current fitness level. This will not only help you set realistic goals but also allow you to choose activities that align with your abilities. Start by reflecting on your daily routine. Are you active or mostly sedentary? Can you walk a short distance without feeling fatigued? Do you have any existing health conditions that might affect your ability to exercise?

To get a more formal assessment, consider using the following simple tests:

- Walking Test: Measure how far you can walk comfortably in 6 minutes. This will give you a baseline of your cardiovascular endurance.
- Chair Stand Test: Sit in a sturdy chair and stand up without using your hands. Count how many times you can do this in 30 seconds. This test gauges leg strength and stability.
- Balance Test: Stand on one leg for as long as you can. This test will help you understand your balance and stability, which are crucial for aerobic activities.

Consider the story of Ruth, an 80-year-old who decided it was time to improve her fitness. After assessing her abilities, she discovered she could walk for about 10 minutes at a time before needing a break. Armed with this knowledge, she set a goal to gradually increase her walking time, which provided her with both direction and motivation.

Consulting with a Doctor Before Starting

Before starting any exercise program, especially if you have existing health concerns or haven't been active for a while, consulting with your doctor is paramount. A healthcare professional can assess your overall health, recommend suitable exercises, and identify any limitations you should be aware of.

For example, if you have a history of heart problems or joint issues, your doctor may suggest specific modifications to ensure you can exercise safely. By having this conversation, you can embark on your fitness journey with confidence, knowing that you are taking the right steps for your health.

After receiving the green light from her doctor, Helen, a 72-year-old grandmother, felt empowered. Her doctor not only approved her plans for low-impact aerobics but also provided tailored advice on heart rate monitoring during workouts. This guidance helped Helen feel secure in her choices and motivated her to start exercising regularly.

Essential Warm-Up Exercises for Seniors

Warming up is a vital component of any exercise routine, particularly for seniors. A good warm-up increases blood flow to your muscles, raises your heart rate gradually, and prepares your body for more strenuous activity. Here are some effective warm-up exercises that seniors can incorporate before their aerobic workouts:

1. Gentle Marching: Stand tall and march in place, lifting your knees gently. Do this for 3–5 minutes to get your blood circulating.

2. Arm Circles: Extend your arms out to the side and make small circles, gradually increasing the size of the circles. This helps to loosen up your shoulders.

3. Side Leg Raises: Hold onto a chair or counter for balance and lift one leg out to the side, then return it to the ground. Alternate legs for 10 repetitions each.

4. Torso Twists: Stand with your feet shoulder-width apart and gently twist your upper body from side to side. This promotes flexibility in your spine and warms up your core.

After warming up, many seniors find they are more energized and ready to tackle their aerobic exercises. Take the case of David, who found that a few minutes of warm-up significantly improved his performance. By integrating simple movements into his routine, he not only felt more prepared but also enjoyed the experience more.

Common Mistakes to Avoid in Senior Aerobics

Starting a new exercise program can sometimes lead to mistakes that might hinder progress or cause injury. Being aware of these pitfalls will help you avoid them:

1. Skipping the Warm-Up: Neglecting to warm up can lead to injuries, as your muscles aren't prepared for the activity ahead.

2. Pushing Too Hard, Too Fast: It's tempting to dive into intense workouts, but this can lead to burnout or injury. Start slow and gradually increase your intensity.

3. Ignoring Pain: While some discomfort is normal when starting a new exercise, sharp or persistent pain is a warning sign. Listen to your body and adjust accordingly.

4. Neglecting Hydration: Staying hydrated is crucial, especially during physical activity. Always drink water before, during, and after your workouts.

5. Not Having Fun: Exercise should be enjoyable! If you dread your workouts, you're less likely to stick with them. Find activities that excite you.

When Martha, a 76-year-old, first started her aerobic journey, she was eager to make up for lost time. However, she quickly learned that her enthusiasm led her to overdo it. After experiencing some discomfort, she decided to slow down and focus on what felt good. This shift allowed her to appreciate her workouts and incorporate fun elements, like dancing, into her routine.

The Role of Mobility and Flexibility in Aerobic Readiness

Mobility and flexibility play crucial roles in preparing your body for aerobic exercises. Improved mobility allows for better movement patterns, while flexibility reduces the risk of injury. Simple stretching exercises can significantly enhance both.

Consider adding stretches like hamstring stretches, calf stretches, and shoulder stretches into your routine. Engaging in activities like yoga or tai chi can also improve mobility and flexibility while providing a gentle introduction to aerobic movements.

For instance, Lily, a 68-year-old yoga enthusiast, found that practicing gentle stretches before her walks made a significant difference. She could stride more comfortably and confidently, transforming her walks into joyful excursions rather than mere exercise.

Getting started with aerobics for seniors is an empowering journey that can lead to a healthier, more vibrant life. By assessing your fitness level, consulting with a doctor, warming up properly, avoiding common mistakes, and prioritizing mobility and flexibility, you set yourself up for success.

As we move forward in this book, you will discover a variety of aerobic exercises and routines tailored to meet your unique needs. Embrace this opportunity to enhance your well-being and connect with the joy of movement. Let's take the next step together, building a foundation for a healthier and more active lifestyle!

CHAPTER 3

SAFE AND EASY-TO-FOLLOW AEROBIC EXERCISES FOR SENIORS

As we venture deeper into the world of aerobics, it's essential to focus on exercises that are safe, effective, and enjoyable for seniors. This chapter will explore low-impact aerobics, walking, chair exercises, water workouts, dancing, and how to modify these activities to suit your individual needs. These activities not only enhance cardiovascular health but also bring joy and connection to the process of staying fit.

Low-Impact Aerobics: What Makes Them Ideal for Seniors?

Low-impact aerobics are designed to minimize the stress on joints while still providing an effective cardiovascular workout. This makes them particularly suitable for seniors, who may experience joint pain or stiffness. Low-impact exercises allow for a gentle approach to fitness, promoting mobility, endurance, and overall well-being.

Imagine Margaret, a 74-year-old grandmother who loves to garden but struggles with knee pain. She discovered low-impact aerobics through a local class that emphasized smooth, controlled movements. By participating in these sessions, Margaret not only strengthened her cardiovascular health but also noticed a significant reduction in her knee discomfort. The combination of aerobic exercise and joint-friendly movements made her gardening more enjoyable, reminding her that staying active can be a delightful experience.

Walking Aerobics: A Simple Way to Get Moving

Walking is one of the easiest and most accessible forms of aerobic exercise, making it an excellent choice for seniors. Not only does it require no special equipment, but it can be done almost anywhere inside, outside, or even in place. Walking aerobics takes this simple activity a step further by incorporating variations such as arm movements, changes in pace, or incorporating hills to enhance the workout.

Samantha, a 70-year-old retiree, found that incorporating walking aerobics into her routine transformed her daily strolls into invigorating sessions. She began by walking around her neighborhood, swinging her arms to increase intensity. As her endurance grew, she added intervals of faster walking and even invited friends to join her, turning her exercise time into a social occasion. This simple change helped Samantha maintain her motivation and reinforced the idea that fitness can be fun.

Chair Aerobics for Seniors with Limited Mobility

For seniors with limited mobility or those recovering from injuries, chair aerobics offer a fantastic alternative to traditional exercises. These workouts allow participants to engage in aerobic movements while seated, making them safe and accessible. Chair aerobics can improve cardiovascular health, flexibility, and strength without the risk of falling.

Consider the story of Carl, an 82-year-old who had undergone hip surgery. Determined to regain his strength, he joined a chair aerobics class at his local community center. The class provided a variety of seated exercises, from arm lifts to seated marches, enabling him to work out without putting stress on his healing hip. As he progressed, Carl not only built strength but also developed friendships with fellow participants, highlighting how social connections can enhance the exercise experience.

Water Aerobics: Gentle on Joints, Great for the Heart

Water aerobics is another exceptional option for seniors seeking a low-impact workout. The buoyancy of water reduces the impact on joints, allowing for a more comfortable and supportive exercise environment. These classes often include a mix of cardiovascular and strength-training exercises, making them an effective way to enhance fitness without the discomfort associated with traditional workouts.

Let's look at how Betty, a vibrant 75-year-old, discovered water aerobics after struggling with arthritis in her knees. She initially hesitated to try a class, fearing it might be too challenging. However, once she took the plunge, she found herself floating effortlessly, moving freely without pain. The instructor guided her through a series of fun, engaging exercises that not only strengthened her muscles but also improved her endurance. As Betty continued to attend classes, she discovered a supportive community of fellow participants, enhancing her social life and fitness journey.

Dancing as an Aerobic Exercise for Fun and Fitness

Dancing is a delightful way to combine aerobic exercise with enjoyment. It's an excellent choice for seniors because it allows for creativity and self-expression while promoting cardiovascular health. Whether it's ballroom dancing, line dancing, or Zumba Gold, there are numerous styles to choose from that cater to various interests and abilities.

Take the inspiring example of Ellen, a lively 68-year-old who had always loved dancing but felt she had lost her groove over the years. She joined a local dance class tailored for seniors and was thrilled to rediscover her passion for movement. The infectious music, along with the friendly faces around her, made each session feel less like a workout and more like a celebration. Dancing not only helped Ellen maintain her fitness but also lifted her spirits, showing that exercise can be a joyful experience.

How to Modify Exercises for Your Needs and Limitations

Understanding that everyone has unique needs and limitations is essential when it comes to aerobics for seniors. Modifications can ensure that exercises remain safe and effective, allowing everyone to participate according to their abilities.

For instance, if a specific movement feels uncomfortable, consider making small adjustments:

- Reduce Range of Motion: If reaching overhead causes discomfort, focus on exercises that involve a smaller range of motion, such as side lifts at shoulder height.
- Slow Down the Pace: If you're struggling to keep up with the tempo of a workout, slow down the movements. Quality over quantity is key in exercise.
- Use Support: Utilize a chair or wall for balance when performing standing exercises, allowing you to focus on the movements without fear of falling.
- Listen to Your Body: Always pay attention to how your body responds to different exercises. If something doesn't feel right, modify or skip that movement.

Consider Jack, a 76-year-old with limited flexibility due to past injuries. He attended a low-impact aerobics class but found that certain exercises were challenging. After speaking with his instructor, Jack learned how to modify the movements to better suit his needs, ensuring he could still enjoy the class while exercising safely. The support and understanding he received empowered him to continue participating and enjoy the camaraderie of the group.

Safe and easy-to-follow aerobic exercises can significantly enhance the quality of life for seniors. Whether it's low-impact aerobics, walking, chair workouts, water exercises, or dancing, the options are diverse and adaptable to individual needs.

As you explore these activities, remember that fitness is not just about physical health; it's about joy, connection, and the opportunity to celebrate movement. In the upcoming chapters, we will delve deeper into creating personalized routines and discovering how to integrate these exercises into your daily life. Let's continue this journey toward a healthier, happier you, one step at a time!

CHAPTER 4

AEROBIC ROUTINES TO BOOST HEART HEALTH

As we continue our journey into the world of aerobics, it's essential to focus on the heart, the vital organ that fuels our bodies and keeps us active. This chapter will explore cardiovascular exercises tailored for seniors, present specific workout plans designed to promote heart health, emphasize the importance of consistency, and guide you on safely monitoring your heart rate during exercise. Each of these elements is crucial for enhancing your cardiovascular health and overall well-being.

Cardio Exercises for a Healthy Heart

Cardiovascular exercises, or cardio, play a pivotal role in maintaining heart health, especially as we age. These exercises strengthen the heart muscle, improve circulation, and help manage weight, blood pressure, and cholesterol levels. The beauty of cardio is its versatility; there are numerous ways to get your heart pumping.

Consider light jogging, brisk walking, swimming, or cycling. For seniors, low-impact activities like walking or water aerobics are often the most beneficial, as they reduce stress on the joints while still providing an effective workout.

Take the story of George, an 80-year-old retiree. After a health scare prompted him to take his heart health seriously, he turned to walking. Each morning, George would walk through his neighborhood, gradually increasing his pace and distance. Over time, he noticed not just improvements in his heart health, but also an enhanced sense of vitality. The regular walks became a cherished part of his day, allowing him to connect with nature and his community while investing in his health.

Senior-Specific Aerobic Workout Plans for Heart Health

Creating a structured aerobic workout plan tailored to seniors can significantly enhance heart health. Here are a few examples of simple, senior-specific workout plans that incorporate various forms of aerobic exercise:

1. Walking Routine:

- Warm-Up: 5–10 minutes of gentle marching in place or light stretching.
- Main Workout: 20–30 minutes of brisk walking. Start with a comfortable pace and gradually increase speed for the last 5–10 minutes.
- Cool Down: 5–10 minutes of slow walking followed by stretching.

2. Chair Aerobics Routine:

- Warm-Up: Seated arm circles and torso twists for 5 minutes.
- Main Workout: 15–20 minutes of exercises like seated leg lifts, seated marches, and overhead arm raises.
- Cool Down: Gentle stretching while seated for 5–10 minutes.

3. Water Aerobics Routine

- Warm-Up: 5–10 minutes of gentle movements in the water, like leg swings and arm circles.
- Main Workout: 20–30 minutes of water jogging, arm exercises with water weights, and gentle resistance movements.
- Cool Down: Slow, gentle stretches in the water for 5–10 minutes.

Regularly following these plans will contribute to improved cardiovascular health while promoting overall strength and mobility. Sarah, a 72-year-old grandmother, embraced a walking routine that helped her lose weight and feel more energetic. She noticed a significant drop in her blood pressure and cholesterol levels, which motivated her to maintain her new active lifestyle.

The Importance of Consistency in Heart Health Improvement

While starting an aerobic routine is a vital step, consistency is the key to reaping the full benefits for heart health. Engaging in regular aerobic exercise aiming for at least 150 minutes of moderate-intensity activity each week can lead to substantial improvements in cardiovascular function and overall well-being.

Consider the experience of Tom, a 76-year-old who initially struggled to maintain a regular exercise routine. After joining a local exercise group, he realized that having a set schedule and working out alongside others made it easier to stay committed. The friendships he formed and the accountability of group workouts helped him stick to his plan, leading to remarkable improvements in his heart health over time. Tom's success story is a powerful reminder that consistency can transform your health journey.

Monitoring Your Heart Rate: How to Do It Safely During Exercise

Understanding how to monitor your heart rate is crucial for safe and effective aerobic exercise. Keeping track of your heart rate helps ensure you're exercising within a safe range, maximizing the benefits while minimizing risks.

Here's how to do it safely:

1. Know Your Target Heart Rate: For most seniors, a target heart rate of 50-70% of your maximum heart rate is ideal for moderate-intensity exercise. To estimate your maximum heart rate, subtract your age from 220. For example, if you're 70 years old, your estimated maximum heart rate is 150 beats per minute (BPM). Therefore, your target heart rate during exercise would be approximately 75-105 BPM.

2. Use the Talk Test: A simple way to gauge your exercise intensity is the "talk test." You should be able to hold a conversation while exercising, but not sing. If you can't speak comfortably, you may be working too hard.

3. Check Your Pulse: You can manually check your pulse by placing your index and middle fingers on the inside of your wrist or the side of your neck. Count the beats for 15 seconds and multiply by four to get your BPM.

4. Use Technology: Consider using a heart rate monitor or fitness tracker to keep an eye on your heart rate during workouts. Many devices provide real-time feedback, making it easier to stay within your target range.

Claire, a 69-year-old fitness enthusiast, started tracking her heart rate during her walking sessions. Initially, she felt unsure about her intensity levels, but with a simple heart rate monitor, she gained confidence in her workouts. This newfound awareness allowed her to adjust her pace as needed and ultimately led to significant improvements in her fitness and heart health.

Aerobic routines designed to boost heart health are essential for seniors seeking to maintain an active lifestyle. Through cardio exercises, tailored workout plans, consistency, and proper heart rate monitoring, you can enhance your cardiovascular fitness and overall well-being.

As we move forward in this book, we will explore more advanced techniques for personalizing your aerobic routines and integrating these practices into your daily life. Remember, each step you take toward heart health is a step toward a more vibrant and fulfilling life. Let's continue this journey together, ensuring that our hearts remain strong and our spirits high!

CHAPTER 5

BUILDING ENDURANCE THROUGH AEROBICS

Building endurance is one of the most rewarding aspects of participating in aerobic exercise, particularly for seniors. This chapter will delve into how aerobic activity enhances stamina, the long-term benefits of improved endurance for daily life, tips for gradually increasing exercise intensity, strategies for avoiding burnout, and inspiring success stories of seniors who have transformed their endurance through aerobic routines.

How Aerobic Exercise Improves Stamina

Aerobic exercise primarily focuses on activities that increase your heart rate and breathing over an extended period, such as walking, swimming, or cycling. As you engage in these activities, your body becomes more efficient at using oxygen, which is key to building stamina. This process involves strengthening your heart, lungs, and muscles, allowing you to perform daily tasks with greater ease.

Take the story of Eleanor, a 75-year-old who once found climbing stairs exhausting. After committing to a regular aerobic routine that included brisk walking and dancing, she noticed remarkable changes. Not only could she climb stairs with newfound vigor, but she also found herself more energetic during her daily activities. The consistent aerobic exercise enhanced her stamina and improved her overall quality of life, demonstrating the transformative power of aerobic fitness.

Long-Term Benefits of Endurance for Daily Activities

Improved endurance through aerobic exercise significantly enhances daily life. With better stamina, simple tasks like grocery shopping, gardening, or playing with grandchildren become less daunting and more enjoyable. Seniors often report feeling more energized and less fatigued throughout the day, allowing for greater participation in activities they love.

For instance, think of Samuel, a 70-year-old grandfather who used to struggle with playing catch with his grandchildren. After a year of consistent aerobic workouts, he discovered that he could easily keep up with the kids during their games. His increased endurance not only brought joy to his family but also strengthened the bonds they shared through play.

In addition to enhancing day-to-day activities, building endurance can also lead to improved mental well-being. The more active seniors feel, the better their mood tends to be. The endorphins released during aerobic exercise contribute to reduced feelings of anxiety and depression, providing an uplifting sense of achievement that resonates beyond physical capabilities.

Tips for Gradually Increasing Aerobic Intensity

When it comes to building endurance, it's crucial to approach intensity gradually. Sudden changes can lead to injury or burnout, hindering your progress. Here are some practical tips for safely ramping up your aerobic intensity:

1. **Start Slow**: If you're new to aerobic exercise, begin with shorter sessions around 15-20 minutes and gradually build up to 30-60 minutes. This allows your body to adapt without overwhelming it.

2. **Increase Duration First**: Focus on extending the length of your workouts before increasing the intensity. For instance, if you typically walk for 20 minutes, aim to walk for 25 minutes next week before adding more speed.

3. **Incorporate Intervals**: As you build confidence, introduce short bursts of higher intensity within your workouts. For example, if you're walking, try brisk walking for one

minute followed by a two-minute recovery pace. This technique can enhance your cardiovascular fitness without the risk of pushing too hard too quickly.

4. Listen to Your Body: Pay attention to how your body responds to changes in intensity. If you feel excessively fatigued or experience pain, dial back your efforts and allow yourself time to recover.

5. Set Realistic Goals: Establish specific, achievable goals for your endurance journey. This could involve completing a certain number of workouts each week or gradually increasing your walking distance. Celebrate your achievements, no matter how small.

After adopting these strategies, Linda, a 68-year-old retiree, felt empowered to gradually increase her aerobic intensity. She started with leisurely walks and, through patience and dedication, transformed her routine into brisk walking and light jogging. Linda's persistence paid off as she completed a local charity walk, feeling accomplished and inspired to continue her journey.

Avoiding Burnout: Rest and Recovery Strategies

While building endurance is exciting, it's equally important to prioritize rest and recovery to prevent burnout. Overtraining can lead to physical fatigue, increased risk of injury, and decreased motivation. Here are some strategies to incorporate recovery into your routine:

1. Schedule Rest Days: Plan regular rest days into your week to allow your body to recover. For example, if you exercise five days a week, consider taking two days for gentle stretching or leisure activities instead of vigorous workouts.

2. Incorporate Variety: To keep things fresh, mix different types of aerobic activities into your routine. This prevents monotony and allows for active recovery. You might alternate walking, swimming, and dancing throughout the week.

3. Prioritize Sleep: Ensure you're getting enough quality sleep each night, as it plays a crucial role in recovery. Aim for 7-9 hours of restorative sleep to support your body's healing processes.

4. Stay Hydrated and Nourished: Proper hydration and nutrition are vital for recovery. Focus on a balanced diet rich in fruits, vegetables, lean proteins, and whole grains to fuel your body effectively.

5. Practice Mindfulness: Incorporate mindfulness practices such as meditation or deep breathing exercises to manage stress. This can help rejuvenate your mind and body, enhancing your overall well-being.

After following these recovery strategies, Joseph, a 74-year-old avid walker, found that he could enjoy his workouts without feeling drained. By respecting his body's need for rest, he maintained a consistent and enjoyable routine, ultimately leading to a more fulfilling exercise experience.

Success Stories: Seniors Who've Improved Endurance Through Aerobics

The power of aerobics to improve endurance is reflected in the inspiring stories of many seniors who have transformed their lives through consistent exercise.

Maria, a 71-year-old woman who faced mobility challenges after a knee injury, turned to water aerobics for support. With determination and a tailored routine, Maria gradually built her endurance. Over time, she could walk longer distances on land and even hike with her family, a passion she thought she had lost forever.

Henry, a 79-year-old retired teacher, discovered a newfound passion for dance classes. At first, he hesitated due to self-doubt, but he embraced the challenge. His weekly dance sessions not only improved his endurance but also fostered friendships with fellow dancers. Henry's journey reflects how stepping outside your comfort zone can lead to remarkable growth.

These stories of resilience and transformation are a testament to the impact of aerobic exercise on seniors' endurance. Each of these individuals has shown that it's never too late to embark on a fitness journey, and that with perseverance, the rewards can be profound.

Building endurance through aerobics is a powerful endeavor that offers countless benefits for seniors. As you enhance your stamina, daily activities become more manageable, and your overall quality of life improves. Remember to approach your aerobic journey with patience, gradually increasing intensity while prioritizing rest and recovery.

With the stories and strategies shared in this chapter, you have the tools to embark on a fulfilling path toward greater endurance. In the next chapters, we will explore how to create personalized aerobic routines and celebrate the joy of movement in your daily life. Together, let's embrace the journey toward building stamina and vitality, ensuring each step forward is a step toward a brighter, more energetic future!

CHAPTER 6

ENERGY-BOOSTING AEROBIC EXERCISES FOR SENIORS

As we age, maintaining energy levels can often feel like an uphill battle. Whether it's the daily demands of life or the natural effects of aging, many seniors struggle with fatigue. However, the good news is that aerobic exercise can be a powerful antidote to low energy levels. This chapter explores how aerobic activity combats fatigue, enhances sleep and mood, introduces short-burst exercises for quick energy boosts, and offers nutritional tips to sustain energy throughout your workouts.

Aerobic Exercise for Combating Fatigue and Improving Energy

Engaging in regular aerobic exercise is a proven way to combat fatigue. While it may seem counterintuitive, how can expending energy lead to increased energy? The science behind it is compelling. Aerobic activities stimulate circulation, delivering oxygen and nutrients to your muscles, which can significantly enhance overall vitality.

Take the story of Doris, an 82-year-old who found herself feeling tired and sluggish after retirement. She decided to join a local walking group. At first, Doris struggled to keep pace, but as she continued to walk regularly, she noticed a remarkable change. With each step, her energy levels began to rise. By incorporating aerobic exercise into her routine, Doris transformed her fatigue into a zest for life. She found joy not just in walking but also in the companionship of her fellow walkers, and her mood noticeably improved.

Incorporating just 30 minutes of moderate aerobic activity most days of the week can significantly reduce feelings of tiredness and increase overall energy levels. This isn't just about physical health; it's also about mental well-being. The endorphins released during exercise create a natural boost in mood, making daily activities more enjoyable and fulfilling.

How Regular Activity Promotes Better Sleep and Mood

A vital aspect of maintaining high energy levels is ensuring good quality sleep. Interestingly, regular aerobic exercise is linked to improved sleep patterns. When you engage in physical activity, your body experiences a natural drop in temperature after exercising, which signals that it's time to rest. This process helps you fall asleep faster and enjoy deeper sleep cycles.

Consider the experience of Gary, a 76-year-old man who often found himself tossing and turning at night. After he began a routine of low-impact aerobics, including swimming and gentle cycling, he noticed that he was sleeping more soundly. The combination of exercise and improved sleep quality gave him the energy boost he craved during the day.

Moreover, physical activity has been shown to alleviate symptoms of anxiety and depression, which can contribute to feelings of fatigue. For seniors, feeling emotionally balanced is crucial for maintaining energy levels. When you exercise regularly, you're not just improving your physical health; you're also nurturing your mental and emotional well-being.

Short-Burst Aerobic Exercises for an Energy Boost

Short-burst aerobic exercises are a fantastic way to elevate energy levels, especially when you need a quick pick-me-up. These exercises require minimal time commitment but can be incredibly effective at revving up your heart rate and boosting your energy. Here are a few easy-to-follow examples:

1. Marching in Place: Stand tall and march in place for 2-5 minutes. Swing your arms and raise your knees to increase intensity. This simple move gets your blood flowing and can be done anywhere, whether at home or in a community center.

2. Jumping Jacks (Modified): If jumping isn't an option, try side-stepping while raising your arms above your head. Do this for 30 seconds to 1 minute. It's a great way to engage your entire body without putting too much stress on your joints.

3. High Knees: Stand with feet hip-width apart and lift one knee toward your chest, then alternate with the other knee. Aim for 30 seconds to a minute of this activity. It's an excellent way to elevate your heart rate quickly.

4. Dancing: Turn on your favorite tunes and dance! Whether it's a slow waltz or a lively jig, dancing is an enjoyable way to incorporate aerobic exercise. Even just 5-10 minutes can lift your spirits and energize your day.

5. Chair Aerobics: For those with limited mobility, chair aerobics can be a fantastic option. Simply sitting in a sturdy chair, raise your arms, tap your feet, or perform seated leg lifts for a few minutes to get your blood flowing.

These short-burst exercises can be strategically incorporated into your daily routine. Whether you're feeling sluggish mid-afternoon or need a wake-up call after a long day, these quick workouts can effectively boost your energy levels and improve your overall mood.

Nutritional Tips for Sustaining Energy During Workouts

While aerobic exercise is a powerful energy booster, proper nutrition is equally vital for sustaining that energy during workouts. Here are some nutritional tips to help you maintain your vitality:

1. Stay Hydrated: Dehydration can lead to fatigue, so it's essential to drink plenty of water throughout the day. Aim for at least 8-10 cups of water, and consider hydrating before, during, and after your workouts.

2. Fuel with Whole Foods: Focus on a balanced diet rich in whole grains, lean proteins, healthy fats, and a variety of fruits and vegetables. These foods provide the essential nutrients needed to support your energy levels. For example, oatmeal topped with berries makes a great pre-workout snack.

3. Eat Small, Frequent Meals: Rather than consuming three large meals a day, consider eating smaller, nutrient-dense snacks throughout the day. This can help stabilize your blood sugar levels and provide a steady source of energy. Nut butter on whole grain crackers or yogurt with fruit are great options.

4. Timing Matters: Fuel your body with carbohydrates about 30 minutes before your workout. Foods like bananas, toast with peanut butter, or a small smoothie can provide the energy needed to power through your aerobic exercises.

5. Post-Workout Recovery: After exercising, prioritize recovery with a snack that combines protein and carbohydrates. A small protein shake, a handful of nuts, or a piece of fruit with cheese can help replenish your energy stores and aid in muscle recovery.

Take the example of Ellen, a 70-year-old who struggled to find the energy to complete her workouts. After consulting a nutritionist, she started incorporating whole foods and hydration strategies into her routine. With a balanced diet and proper hydration, Ellen felt more energized during her workouts, allowing her to push through and enjoy her aerobic sessions.

Aerobic exercise can be a game-changer in combating fatigue and boosting energy levels for seniors. By engaging in regular activity, you not only improve your physical health but also enhance your mood and promote better sleep. The introduction of short-burst exercises can provide immediate energy boosts, while thoughtful nutrition helps sustain that energy for optimal performance.

As you continue your journey through this book, remember that every step you take toward improved fitness and health can lead to a more vibrant, energetic life. Let the stories and strategies shared here inspire you to embrace the invigorating world of aerobic exercise. Together, let's harness the power of movement to unlock a future filled with energy and vitality!

CHAPTER 7

GROUP AEROBIC CLASSES FOR SENIORS

Engaging in aerobic exercise doesn't have to be a solitary journey. In fact, one of the most enjoyable and effective ways to stay active is through group classes tailored specifically for seniors. This chapter delves into the many benefits of social fitness, explores the variety of group aerobic classes available, and offers practical advice on how to find or create local groups. Additionally, we'll look at online and virtual options that can expand your reach and make staying active easier than ever.

Benefits of Social Fitness: Exercising with Others

Social interaction is a crucial component of our overall well-being, especially as we age. Participating in group aerobic classes offers not just physical benefits, but also emotional and social rewards. When seniors exercise together, they foster a sense of community that can combat feelings of isolation and loneliness, which are common challenges for many older adults.

Take the story of Margaret, an 85-year-old widow who had recently moved to a new town. Initially, she felt lonely and disconnected from her new environment. However, when she joined a local senior aerobics class, everything changed. The class provided her with a welcoming space to meet new friends and connect with others who shared her interests. Not only did Margaret find joy in the exercises, but she also formed lasting friendships. Together, they would often grab coffee after class, sharing laughs and stories that enriched her life.

The social aspect of exercising in a group encourages accountability as well. When you know that others are counting on you to show up, it can motivate you to stick to your routine. The encouragement from fellow participants, combined with the camaraderie, can make exercising feel less like a chore and more like a fun, engaging activity.

Types of Group Aerobic Classes Tailored to Seniors

As the fitness industry has grown, so have the options available for senior-focused aerobic classes. Here are some popular types:

1. Low-Impact Aerobics: Designed to minimize stress on joints while providing an effective workout, low-impact aerobics classes focus on movements that are gentle yet effective. They typically include activities like marching, side steps, and arm raises.

2. Chair Aerobics: For seniors with limited mobility, chair aerobics can be a fantastic option. These classes are conducted while seated, allowing participants to engage in gentle movements that improve strength and flexibility without risking falls or injuries.

3. Water Aerobics: Conducted in a pool, water aerobics classes offer buoyancy that reduces strain on joints, making it an excellent choice for seniors. These classes typically include resistance exercises that can help build strength while providing a refreshing environment.

4. Dance Aerobics: Dance-inspired classes, such as Zumba Gold or line dancing, combine music with movement, making workouts fun and lively. These classes often encourage participants to express themselves through dance, creating a joyful atmosphere.

5. Tai Chi and Qigong: While not traditional aerobic exercises, these classes focus on gentle, flowing movements that improve balance, coordination, and overall body awareness. They promote mindfulness and relaxation, making them an excellent complement to more vigorous aerobic workouts.

6. Circuit Training: Some classes incorporate circuit training, where participants move through various stations that combine aerobic and strength-training exercises. This variety keeps workouts fresh and engaging while offering a full-body experience.

How to Find or Create a Local Senior Aerobics Group

Finding the right group can greatly enhance your exercise experience. Here are some practical tips on how to locate local senior aerobics classes:

1. Community Centers: Many towns and cities have community centers that offer a variety of fitness classes specifically designed for seniors. Check their schedules or visit in person to explore options.

2. Fitness Studios and Gyms: Some fitness studios and gyms cater specifically to older adults, offering specialized classes. Inquire about any senior-friendly programs they may have

3. Senior Centers and Assisted Living Facilities: These facilities often provide organized exercise classes or can connect you with local resources for group workouts.

4. Local Parks and Recreation Departments: Many municipalities offer fitness classes in local parks. These classes can be a wonderful way to enjoy the outdoors while staying active.

5. Social Media and Community Boards: Online platforms like Facebook often have community groups where local events and activities are shared. Search for senior fitness groups in your area to discover classes and meet-ups.

If you can't find a group that meets your needs, consider creating your own! Here's how:

- Gather Friends: Reach out to friends, neighbors, or fellow church members who might be interested in exercising together. Having a small group can create a supportive environment.

- Choose a Venue: Decide on a location that's convenient and comfortable, such as someone's home, a community center, or even a local park.

- Design a Schedule: Determine a regular meeting time that works for everyone, whether it's once a week or several times a week. Consistency is key to maintaining engagement.

- Select Activities: Collaboratively choose the types of exercises you want to do. You could follow online videos, create a playlist for dance classes, or even invite a local instructor to guide you.

Online and Virtual Aerobic Classes for Seniors

In today's digital age, online and virtual classes have made exercising more accessible than ever. These options allow seniors to participate in aerobic exercises from the comfort of their own homes, providing flexibility and convenience. Here's how to explore this option:

1. YouTube Channels: There are numerous fitness channels dedicated to senior-friendly workouts. Search for terms like "senior aerobics," "chair exercises," or "water aerobics" to find videos that suit your needs.

2. Streaming Services: Many fitness platforms offer subscription-based services with a variety of classes. You can explore different styles of aerobic exercise and select what resonates most with you.

3. Virtual Community Groups: Join online communities focused on senior fitness. These groups often share virtual class schedules, fitness challenges, and motivational content, creating a sense of community even from a distance.

4. Local Classes Going Virtual: Many local fitness studios and community centers have adapted to the pandemic by offering online classes. Check with your local facilities to see if they provide virtual options.

5. Fitness Apps: Consider downloading apps specifically designed for seniors. These apps may offer guided workouts, nutrition tips, and community features to connect with other seniors interested in fitness.

Take inspiration from Bill, a 78-year-old who discovered virtual classes during the pandemic. Initially skeptical, he soon found that participating in live-streamed aerobics classes allowed him to stay active while connecting with others from his living room. Bill enjoyed the energy of the instructors and even made friends through the online platform. As a bonus, he could replay classes whenever he wanted, ensuring he never missed a workout.

Group aerobic classes offer seniors a unique opportunity to enhance their physical health while cultivating meaningful social connections. The benefits of exercising with others extend far beyond physical fitness; they create a sense of belonging and camaraderie that enriches lives. Whether you choose to join an established class or create your own group, the key is to find an activity that you enjoy and that motivates you to stay active.

As you continue your journey toward fitness, remember that community plays a vital role in keeping you engaged and inspired. With the right support and resources, you can embrace the joy of movement and foster lasting connections with others. So gather your friends, explore local options, or hop into a virtual class, and let the power of group aerobics elevate your fitness experience!

CHAPTER 8

AEROBICS FOR SENIORS WITH CHRONIC CONDITIONS

As we age, the likelihood of living with chronic conditions increases, which can present unique challenges when it comes to maintaining an active lifestyle. However, engaging in aerobic exercise can significantly improve quality of life for seniors with conditions like arthritis, diabetes, or osteoporosis. This chapter will explore how to adapt aerobic exercises for those with chronic conditions, focusing on low-impact exercises, special considerations for limited mobility, and how aerobics can complement medical treatments.

Adapting Aerobic Exercises for Seniors with Chronic Conditions

Chronic conditions can influence how seniors approach exercise. Understanding how to adapt aerobic routines is essential for ensuring that they are safe, effective, and enjoyable. Here are some common conditions and adaptations that can be made:

1. Arthritis: Joint pain and stiffness are hallmarks of arthritis, but movement can help alleviate these symptoms. Low-impact exercises, such as swimming or cycling, are excellent options. Margaret, who has rheumatoid arthritis, shares how she found relief in water aerobics. "The buoyancy of the water takes the pressure off my joints," she explains. "I can move freely and feel less pain, all while strengthening my body."

2. Diabetes: For seniors managing diabetes, aerobic exercise can help regulate blood sugar levels and improve insulin sensitivity. Activities like brisk walking or dancing are beneficial. John, a 72-year-old living with type 2 diabetes, highlights his experience, saying, "Since I started attending group classes, my blood sugar levels have stabilized, and I feel more energetic throughout the day."

3. Osteoporosis: Seniors with osteoporosis need to be cautious about high-impact activities that could lead to fractures. However, low-impact aerobics, combined with weight-bearing exercises, can help maintain bone density. Yoga or tai chi can improve balance and flexibility, reducing the risk of falls. Sarah, who has osteoporosis, shares her success: "I was terrified of falling, but after joining a gentle yoga class, I feel much more stable and confident."

Low-Impact Exercises for Heart Disease Management

For seniors with heart disease, aerobic exercise is essential but must be approached with care. Low-impact activities that get the heart rate up without placing excessive strain on the body are ideal. Here are some recommended exercises:

- Walking: One of the simplest and most effective forms of aerobic exercise. It can be done anywhere and at any pace. Starting with short distances and gradually increasing duration is a safe way to build endurance. Helen, a heart disease survivor, says, "Walking in my neighborhood has not only improved my heart health, but it's also a great way to meet neighbors and enjoy the fresh air."
- Stationary Biking: A stationary bike provides an excellent way to elevate the heart rate without the risk of falling. Adjusting the resistance allows for gradual increases in intensity. For Arnold, who has a history of heart issues, biking has become his go-to exercise. "It's low impact, and I can do it while watching my favorite shows," he notes.
- Chair Aerobics: For those who may struggle with traditional exercises, chair aerobics can offer an accessible option that still elevates heart rates. These routines often include seated marching, arm movements, and leg extensions. "I never

thought I could get a good workout from my chair, but it's made a world of difference in how I feel," shares Grace, who uses a chair due to mobility issues.

Exercise Tips for Seniors with Limited Mobility or Chronic Pain

For seniors dealing with limited mobility or chronic pain, exercise may feel daunting. However, adapting routines can make a significant difference in overcoming these barriers:

- Listen to Your Body: Pay attention to pain signals. It's essential to differentiate between discomfort from exertion and pain that indicates injury. Mild soreness is normal, but sharp pain should be a signal to stop.
- Start Slow: Begin with shorter, less intense sessions. As strength and endurance build, gradually increase the duration and intensity. For example, start with 5-10 minutes of gentle movement and slowly work up to 20-30 minutes.
- Modify Movements: Don't hesitate to adapt exercises to fit your comfort level. For instance, instead of jumping jacks, try stepping side to side while raising your arms. Mary, who suffers from chronic back pain, explains, "Modifying exercises helped me feel empowered. I can still move and get my heart pumping without the fear of hurting myself."
- Incorporate Gentle Stretching: Before and after aerobic sessions, include gentle stretches to improve flexibility and reduce muscle tension. This can make a significant difference in how you feel during and after workouts.
- Focus on Breathing: Deep breathing can enhance oxygen flow and help with relaxation during exercise. Practice inhaling deeply through the nose and exhaling through the mouth to promote mindfulness and ease anxiety.

How Aerobics Can Complement Medical Treatment

Aerobics should not be viewed as a substitute for medical treatment, but rather as a complementary approach that can enhance overall health. Engaging in regular aerobic activity can have numerous benefits for seniors dealing with chronic conditions:

1. Enhanced Recovery: Aerobic exercise can speed up recovery times following medical procedures or illnesses. It promotes circulation and can help prevent complications, as seen with Frank, who was encouraged to walk after surgery. "I started small, but now I feel stronger and more capable of getting back to my normal routine," he shares.

2. Improved Mood: Regular exercise has been shown to boost mood and reduce feelings of anxiety and depression. For seniors managing chronic conditions, maintaining mental health is just as important as physical health. Alice, who participates in a weekly dance class, says, "Dancing lifts my spirits. I forget about my worries and just enjoy the moment."

3. Better Communication with Healthcare Providers: Seniors who engage in regular aerobic activity often have more positive interactions with their healthcare teams. They can provide valuable feedback about their symptoms and how their bodies respond to treatment, as explained by Dr. Taylor, a geriatric physician. "When my patients are active, they tend to have better insights into their health, which helps us make informed decisions together."

4. Increased Independence: Maintaining a regular exercise routine can help seniors feel more capable in their daily activities. As they gain strength and endurance, they may find it easier to complete everyday tasks, from grocery shopping to gardening. For David, a once-sedentary senior, this newfound independence has been life-changing. "I can do more for myself now, and it feels incredible," he beams.

Aerobics offers a myriad of benefits for seniors living with chronic conditions. By adapting exercises to fit individual needs and focusing on low-impact activities, seniors can enhance their physical health while managing their conditions. Whether it's through water aerobics, chair workouts, or simple walking routines, the key is to find activities that are enjoyable and safe.

As you embark on this journey, remember that every small step counts. Celebrate your progress, and don't hesitate to seek support from friends, family, or healthcare professionals. By incorporating aerobics into your routine, you can take charge of your health, enhance your quality of life, and rediscover the joy of movement, regardless of the challenges you face.

CHAPTER 9

AEROBIC WORKOUTS FOR THE HOME

In today's fast-paced world, finding the time and means to engage in regular exercise can be challenging, especially for seniors. Fortunately, designing an effective aerobic workout routine at home is not only convenient but can also be tailored to individual needs and preferences. In this chapter, we'll explore how to create a home aerobic workout routine, the minimal equipment you might need, ways to incorporate technology into your fitness regimen, and strategies to balance safety with independence while exercising at home.

How to Design a Home Aerobic Workout Routine

Creating a home aerobic workout routine begins with understanding your fitness level, preferences, and available space. Here's a step-by-step approach to help you get started:

1. Assess Your Space: Take a look around your home and identify a suitable area for exercising. This could be a living room, a spare bedroom, or even a backyard. Ensure the space is free from hazards, like loose rugs or clutter, to create a safe workout environment.

2. Set Goals: Decide what you want to achieve with your aerobic workouts. Are you looking to improve cardiovascular health, lose weight, or simply stay active? Setting specific and achievable goals will help keep you motivated and provide direction for your workouts.

3. Choose Activities: Identify aerobic activities you enjoy and can do at home. This could include walking in place, dancing, chair aerobics, or even using a stationary bike if you have one. The key is to find movements that feel good and are enjoyable.

4. Create a Schedule: Consistency is vital for seeing results. Plan your workouts at specific times during the week, whether it's every morning, a few days a week, or on weekends. Building a routine will make it easier to stick with it.

5. Warm Up and Cool Down: Always include a warm-up to prepare your body for exercise and a cool-down to help it recover afterward. Gentle stretching, light marching in place, or arm circles are great ways to start and finish your workout.

By tailoring your routine to your needs and preferences, you'll not only make exercising at home more enjoyable, but you'll also increase the likelihood of sticking with it.

Minimal Equipment Aerobic Exercises

While many aerobic exercises can be performed without equipment, incorporating minimal equipment can enhance your workouts and add variety. Here are some suggestions:

1. Resistance Bands: These lightweight bands can be used for various aerobic and strength exercises. They're easy to store and can provide resistance during movements, enhancing your workout without straining your joints. For example, you can use bands for seated rows, chest presses, or even leg lifts while seated.

2. Light Weights: A pair of light dumbbells can be beneficial for adding resistance to aerobic workouts. Exercises like arm curls, shoulder presses, and lateral raises can be incorporated into your routine, combining aerobic movements with strength training. Frances, an avid home exerciser, explains, "Using light weights makes me feel stronger, and I can do it all from my living room!"

3. Stability Balls: These large, inflatable balls can improve balance and stability while providing a fun way to engage in aerobic activities. You can sit on the ball while doing upper body movements or use it for stability during exercises like wall squats.

4. Step Platforms: If you have the space, a sturdy step platform can provide an excellent way to add intensity to your workouts. Step-ups and lateral movements on the platform can elevate your heart rate while being gentle on the joints.

5. Fitness Mat: A cushioned mat can make floor exercises more comfortable, whether you're doing stretches, seated workouts, or floor aerobics. It's also easy to roll up and store when not in use.

Using minimal equipment not only enhances your aerobic workouts but also keeps things interesting and allows you to target different muscle groups.

Incorporating Technology: Fitness Apps and Videos for Seniors

In our digital age, technology can serve as a valuable tool in our fitness journeys. Many seniors are discovering the benefits of fitness apps and online videos designed specifically for their age group. Here's how to make the most of these resources:

1. Fitness Apps: Numerous apps cater to seniors, offering guided workouts, tracking tools, and progress monitoring. Apps like "SilverSneakers" provide a wide variety of low-impact exercise routines, while "MyFitnessPal" helps track nutrition and activity. For Emily, who found it challenging to stay motivated, using a fitness app made a world of difference. "I love being able to track my workouts and see how far I've come," she shares.

2. Online Workout Videos: Platforms like YouTube host a plethora of workout videos tailored for seniors. From dance aerobics to gentle yoga sessions, the variety is vast. Look for channels that focus on senior fitness, such as "Hasfit" or "Senior Fitness with Meredith." The visual demonstrations and clear instructions make it easy to follow along at your own pace.

3. Virtual Classes: Many fitness organizations now offer live online classes where you can join a group workout from the comfort of your home. Participating in these classes can foster a sense of community and accountability. Joan, who regularly attends a virtual aerobics class, remarks, "I love seeing familiar faces on the screen. It makes me feel connected, even while exercising at home."

4. Wearable Technology: Devices like fitness trackers can monitor heart rate, steps taken, and calories burned. These insights can help you adjust your workouts based on your progress. Mark, who uses a fitness tracker, appreciates how it motivates him to keep moving. "It's like having a coach on my wrist," he says.

Incorporating technology into your workout routine can enhance motivation, provide guidance, and make exercising more enjoyable.

Balancing Safety and Independence While Exercising at Home

While exercising at home offers convenience, safety is paramount. Here are some strategies to ensure a safe workout environment while maintaining your independence:

1. Establish a Safe Environment: Before starting your workout, ensure your exercise space is clutter-free and well-lit. Remove any potential hazards, like loose cords or unstable furniture, to minimize the risk of falls.

2. Inform Family or Friends: Let someone know your exercise schedule and location in case of emergencies. This simple step can provide peace of mind, especially if you're trying new activities.

3. Use Supportive Footwear: Wearing proper shoes can prevent slips and provide the necessary support for your feet and ankles. Avoid exercising in socks or slippers, as they can increase the risk of falls.

4. Modify When Necessary: Listen to your body and make modifications as needed. If an exercise feels too challenging or causes discomfort, don't hesitate to adjust or switch to a different movement.

5. Know When to Stop: Recognize your body's signals. If you experience any pain or unusual symptoms, stop your workout and rest. It's essential to prioritize your health and well-being.

6. Consider a Buddy System: Exercising with a friend or family member can make workouts more enjoyable and provide an additional layer of safety. You can encourage each other and enjoy shared experiences.

By maintaining safety protocols while enjoying the independence of exercising at home, seniors can create an effective and fulfilling fitness routine.

Designing a home aerobic workout routine empowers seniors to take charge of their health and well-being. By utilizing minimal equipment, incorporating technology, and emphasizing safety, seniors can create an effective exercise regimen that suits their lifestyle and preferences.

Remember, the key to a successful home workout is finding activities you enjoy and sticking with them. Celebrate your progress, no matter how small, and don't hesitate to reach out for support from loved ones or online communities. With commitment and creativity, you can embrace the joy of movement right in the comfort of your home, leading to a healthier, more active life.

CHAPTER 10

MOTIVATION AND OVERCOMING BARRIERS TO EXERCISE

As we age, the decision to stay active can be clouded by a myriad of challenges and excuses. For many seniors, common sentiments such as "I'm too old" or "I'm too tired" can hinder the motivation to engage in aerobic exercises. However, overcoming these barriers is not only possible; it's essential for a healthier, happier life. In this chapter, we'll explore how to tackle common excuses, maintain motivation when exercising alone, set realistic goals, and celebrate the rewarding benefits of regular aerobic activity.

Overcoming Common Excuses

It's easy to dismiss exercise with a variety of excuses, but identifying and reframing these thoughts can pave the way for a more active lifestyle.

1. "I'm Too Old": Aging is often mistakenly associated with a decline in physical capability. In reality, regular aerobic activity can enhance mobility, strength, and overall well-being, regardless of age. Many seniors, like Bob, in their late seventies, have found that starting an exercise routine invigorates their lives. Bob shares, "I used to think I was too old to start exercising. But once I began, I felt more energetic than ever. It's never too late!"

2. "I'm Too Tired": Fatigue can feel overwhelming, especially when energy levels fluctuate. However, physical activity can actually boost energy. Engaging in aerobic exercise releases endorphins, which can elevate mood and combat feelings of fatigue. Lucy, a retiree, often feels tired after a long day, yet she finds that even a short walk recharges her. "I've learned that moving a little can help me feel more awake and alive," she says.

3. "I Don't Have Time": Life can get busy, but finding time for exercise is essential for your health. Consider scheduling workouts like appointments or breaking them into smaller segments throughout the day. Even ten minutes of activity can be beneficial. Carla, a busy grandmother, finds ways to incorporate short bursts of exercise while watching her grandkids. "I'll dance around the living room with them, it's fun, and I don't even realize I'm working out!"

By challenging these excuses and reframing your mindset, you can create opportunities for regular activity.

How to Stay Motivated When Exercising Alone

When exercising alone, it can be easy to lose motivation. Here are some strategies to keep your spirits high and your body moving:

1. Create a Workout Playlist: Music can be a powerful motivator. Compile a playlist of your favorite songs that inspire you to move. Uplifting melodies can make your workout feel more enjoyable and energizing. Martin, who exercises at home, shares, "I love blasting my oldies while I work out. It keeps me motivated and takes me back to happy times!"

2. Join Online Communities: Engaging with others through social media groups or forums focused on senior fitness can help create a sense of community. Sharing experiences, challenges, and successes with like-minded individuals can boost motivation and accountability. Jane, a participant in an online fitness forum, finds encouragement from others: "It feels great to know I'm not alone in this journey."

3. Visualize Your Progress: Keeping a visual reminder of your fitness journey can help maintain motivation. Consider a progress chart, or take before-and-after photos. Celebrating milestones whether it's completing a certain number of workouts or increasing your activity duration can provide a sense of accomplishment.

4. Set a Routine: Establishing a regular schedule for your workouts can make exercise a part of your daily routine. Just like brushing your teeth or having breakfast, prioritize your workout time, and it will become a habit. "I set a specific time each day for my workouts. Once it's on my calendar, I treat it like any important appointment," shares Sarah.

Setting Realistic Goals and Tracking Progress

Goal-setting is crucial for maintaining motivation and making exercise a consistent part of your life. Here's how to set realistic goals and effectively track your progress:

1. SMART Goals: Use the SMART framework Specific, Measurable, Achievable, Relevant, and Time-bound. For example, instead of saying, "I want to exercise more," set a goal like, "I will walk for 20 minutes every day for the next month." This clarity will provide direction and motivation.

2. Break Goals into Smaller Steps: Large goals can be daunting. Break them down into smaller, manageable steps. If your ultimate goal is to walk 30 minutes a day, start with 10 minutes and gradually increase your time each week. Barbara, who followed this method, explains, "Starting small helped me build confidence. Now, I'm walking more than I ever thought I could!"

3. Use a Journal or App: Tracking your workouts in a journal or a fitness app can help you monitor progress and celebrate achievements. Logging your exercises, durations, and how you felt can provide valuable insights and motivation. "Looking back at my journal reminds me of how far I've come," says Gary, a dedicated exerciser.

4. Celebrate Achievements: Acknowledge and celebrate your successes, no matter how small. Whether it's treating yourself to a new workout outfit or indulging in a favorite snack, recognizing your hard work will reinforce your commitment to staying active.

Rewards of Regular Aerobic Exercise: Feeling Better, Living Longer

The benefits of incorporating regular aerobic exercise into your life extend beyond physical fitness. Here are some remarkable rewards that come with staying active:

1. Improved Mood: Exercise is known to enhance mood and reduce symptoms of anxiety and depression. The endorphins released during aerobic activity act as natural mood lifters, leading to a more positive outlook on life.

2. Increased Energy: As discussed earlier, regular movement boosts energy levels. Engaging in aerobic exercise helps combat fatigue, allowing you to enjoy daily activities with greater vigor and enthusiasm.

3. Enhanced Longevity: Research consistently shows that active individuals tend to live longer, healthier lives. Aerobic exercise promotes cardiovascular health, reducing the risk of chronic diseases and improving overall quality of life.

4. Stronger Social Connections: Engaging in group activities or classes fosters social interactions, which are vital for mental and emotional well-being. Connecting with others through exercise can help combat feelings of loneliness and isolation.

5. Greater Independence: Maintaining physical fitness enhances your ability to perform daily activities independently. The more active you are, the more capable you'll feel, which can significantly enhance your quality of life.

Regular aerobic exercise isn't just about the physical benefits; it's about feeling better, living longer, and embracing a fulfilling life.

Overcoming barriers to exercise is essential for seniors seeking to lead healthier, more active lives. By challenging common excuses, finding motivation in solo workouts, setting achievable goals, and celebrating the rewards of regular aerobic exercise, you can transform your perspective on fitness.

Remember, every step you take whether small or significant contributes to your overall well-being. Embrace the journey, stay committed, and celebrate your achievements along the way. By cultivating a positive mindset and prioritizing movement, you'll discover the joy and vitality that comes with an active lifestyle. Your best years can be ahead of you, filled with energy, strength, and endless possibilities.

CONCLUSION

As we reach the end of our exploration into the world of aerobics for seniors, it's essential to reflect on the long-term rewards that come from committing to a more active lifestyle. Engaging in regular aerobic activity offers profound benefits that extend far beyond mere physical fitness. It is a powerful tool for enhancing overall well-being, fostering independence, and improving quality of life.

Reflecting on the Long-Term Rewards of Aerobic Activity

The advantages of maintaining a consistent aerobic routine are well-documented. From improved cardiovascular health to enhanced mood and increased energy levels, these benefits can significantly transform your daily experience. As many of our success stories have shown, seniors who embrace aerobic exercises often report feeling more vibrant and connected to their bodies. For instance, Eleanor, who started a walking program at age 70, noted, "I never thought I could feel this good at my age. I have more energy for my grandkids and feel so much lighter in spirit."

Moreover, the impact of regular aerobic exercise on longevity cannot be overstated. Studies reveal that individuals who remain active are less likely to develop chronic conditions, enabling them to lead healthier, longer lives. Embracing this commitment to aerobic fitness can lead to a cascade of positive changes that enhance not just physical health but emotional and mental resilience as well.

Encouraging Lifelong Commitment to Aerobic Fitness

Incorporating aerobic activity into your daily routine shouldn't feel like a chore; it should be a celebration of movement and vitality. As we age, it's vital to adopt a mindset that values fitness as a lifelong journey rather than a destination. This commitment can foster a deeper connection with our bodies and our overall health.

Consider ways to make exercise enjoyable and meaningful. Join a group class, find a walking buddy, or explore new forms of movement like dance or water aerobics. These experiences not only keep you active but also enhance social connections, which are crucial for emotional health. Remember, the goal is not to be perfect but to be consistent and adapt as your body changes.

Final Thoughts on Adapting Exercises as You Age

Aging is a natural part of life, and with it comes the need to adapt our fitness routines. It's essential to listen to your body and be open to modifying exercises to accommodate your needs and limitations. Whether through low-impact aerobics, chair workouts, or water-based exercises, there are countless options available to help you stay active while respecting your body's signals.

As we conclude, I encourage you to view fitness as a lifelong companion. Your journey in aerobic activity is unique and should reflect your personal preferences and abilities. Each step you take, every class you join, and all the laughter you share with fellow exercisers contribute to your health and happiness.

Appendices

To support your journey into aerobics, here are some helpful resources and plans to guide you:

- Sample Weekly Aerobic Exercise Plan for Beginners: A simple schedule to help you get started with regular aerobic activity tailored for seniors.
- Aerobic Exercises for Seniors with Mobility Challenges: A list of effective exercises designed specifically for those with limited mobility to ensure everyone can participate in fitness.
- Heart Rate Chart for Seniors: A guide to help you monitor your heart rate during exercise, ensuring you stay within safe and effective ranges.
- Resources for Finding Senior Aerobic Classes Online and In-Person: A compilation of resources to help you locate classes and groups that cater to seniors, both virtually and in your community.

In summary, the journey to better health through aerobic exercise is one filled with opportunity, connection, and joy. By embracing this path, you'll not only enhance your physical capabilities but also enrich your life in ways you may never have imagined. Here's to your health, happiness, and the many adventures that await as you continue to move forward!